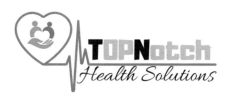

S.H.I.F.T.

Stress & Sleep

Healthy Eating

Intestinal Health

Fitness & Movement

Trust The Process

SHIFT 30-Day Wellness Guide

PAULA RICHARDSON, RN, MSN
FNP-C, AGACNP-BC

S.H.I.F.T. 30-Day Wellness Guide
Copyright © 2024 by Paula Richardson, NP

All rights reserved.

ISBN 979-8-218-49720-0 (printed)

THIS IS ONLY A GUIDE

The complete program kit below can be purchased on our website at Shop.TNHealthsolutions.org

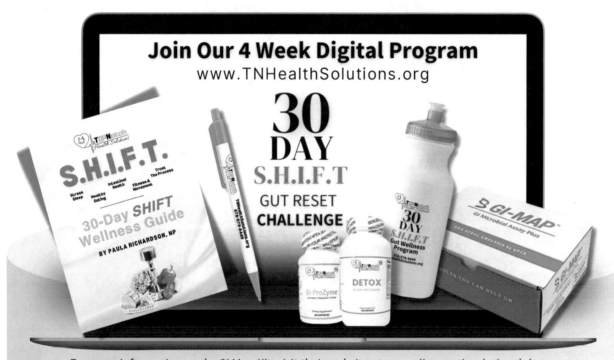

For more information on the GI Map Kit, visit their website at www.diagnosticsolutionslab.com

Limit of Liability/Disclaimer of Warranty
The information shared here is for informational purposes only and should not be considered as medical advice. It is not intended to replace consultation with a qualified healthcare professional. Always seek the advice of your healthcare provider for any medical concerns or questions you may have.

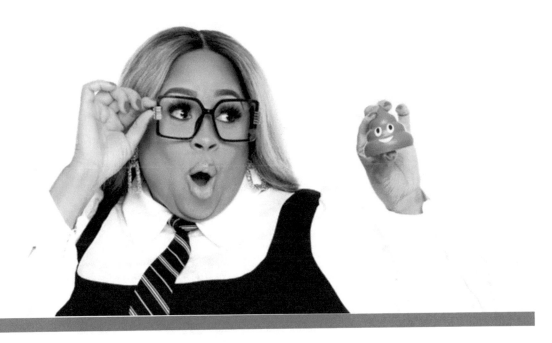

Welcome to
Your S.H.I.F.T.
—

Welcome to S.H.I.F.T., your 30-day wellness guide designed to bring awareness and mindfulness to the essential aspects of your well-being: Sleep & Stress Management, Healthy Eating, Intestinal Health, Fitness & Movement, and Trusting The Process. Embarking on this journey with us means committing to a transformative experience that starts with journaling and habit logging. These practices will heighten your self-awareness and illuminate the areas in need of positive change. By documenting your progress, you cultivate accountability and honesty with yourself, paving the way for a holistic transformation of your overall well-being. Let's begin this empowering journey together.

To shift means to make a change or adjustment, particularly in one's perspective, habits, or approach.

What To Expect
for the next 30-days

1 **Daily Inspirational Affirmations**

2 **Daily Intentional Practices**

3 **Daily Introspection Journaling**

4 **Daily Inscribing of Your Progress**

You have the power to make the SHIFT in your life, transforming your well-being one intentional step at a time. As you embark on this journey, remember to be patient with yourself. Growth and change take time, and each day is an opportunity to progress. Embrace the process with kindness and perseverance, knowing that every effort you make is a step closer to your goals. Trust in your ability to evolve and stay committed to the path ahead. Your journey is unique, and with patience and dedication, you can achieve the transformation you seek.

S.H.I.F.T. *WELLNESS GUIDE*
Transform Your Life with Simple, Holistic Steps

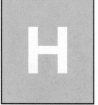

Sleep & Stress
Stress and not getting enough sleep promote unhealthy gut bacteria to grow. Adopting healthy ways to manage stress and promote sleep are very important!

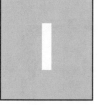

Healthy Eating
Make sure to include whole grains, lean protein, and fiber (5 servings of fruits & vegetables) in each meal at least 80% of the time

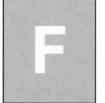

Intestinal Health
Start on our holistic probiotics and the 14 Day System Detox to promote healthy gut bacteria, promote healthy digestion, and decrease inflammation.
Supplements can be purchased on our website at Shop.TNHealthsolutions.org

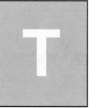

Fitness & Movement
Daily movement is a key aspect to promote a healthy gut. Exercise helps your healthy gut bacteria thrive

Trust the Process
Trust the process! Healing your gut takes time, but every small step counts. Stay patient, consistent, and remember that progress may not always be right away. Your body is working hard to restore balance, so believe the journey, and celebrate each improvement.

Sketch your goals with kindness, remembering that they are fluid and can adapt to your journey's needs.

Explore Our Other Holistic Supplements

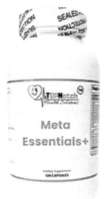

Promoting Metabolic Health starts at the cellular level. Meta Essentials supports metabolic health with the perfect combination of natural herbs that promotes detoxification and energy at the cellular level in addition to essential vitamins and nutrients all in ONE Supplement.

PREVENZYME™ is a special soothing formulation of eight natural digestive enzymes. When we supplement with 8-10 tablets daily, the body will digest 60 grams of fat, 48 grams of protein and 48 grams of carbohydrates. This amount is equal to approximately 1000 calories, which is at least one half the amount an average person consumes in one day.

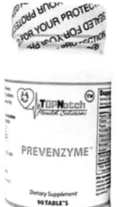

Prevenzyme™ digestive enzymes may provide the following benefits:
• Increases liver and bile function
• Helps to reduce allergies and food sensitivities

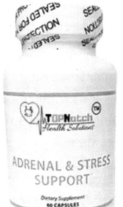

Stress increases cortisol levels that contribute to weight gain. The stress response is designed to support the body needs for a fight or flight response during acute situations.

Chronic low levels of stress on the body causes weight gain and storage of fat...especially in the GUT!!!!What situations stimulated the stress response?

• Lack of Sleep
• Psychological Stress
• Lack of Exercise or too much exercise
• Lack of proper nutrients

Vitamins and Supplements Schedule

> **"I honor the connection between my gut and immune system, supporting overall wellness."**

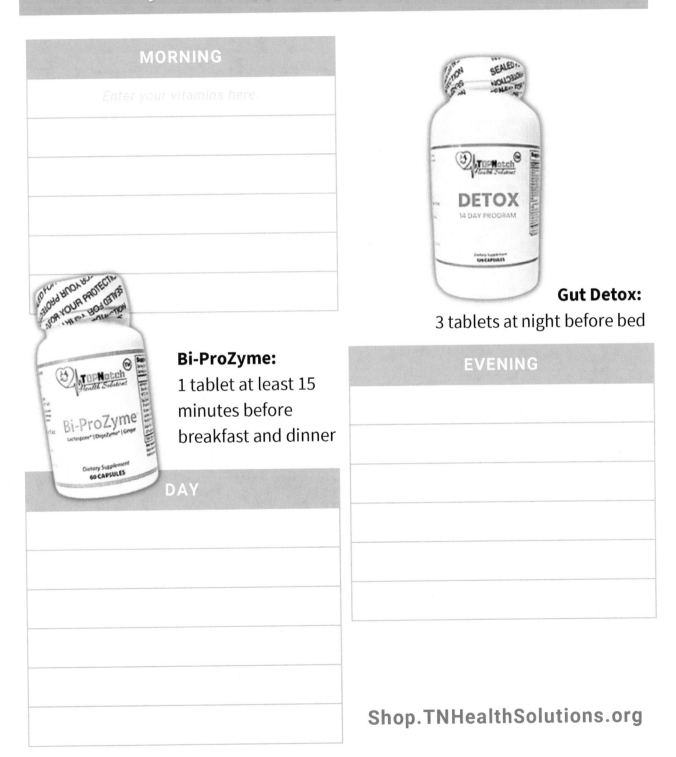

MORNING

Enter your vitamins here.

Gut Detox:

3 tablets at night before bed

Bi-ProZyme:

1 tablet at least 15 minutes before breakfast and dinner

EVENING

DAY

Shop.TNHealthSolutions.org

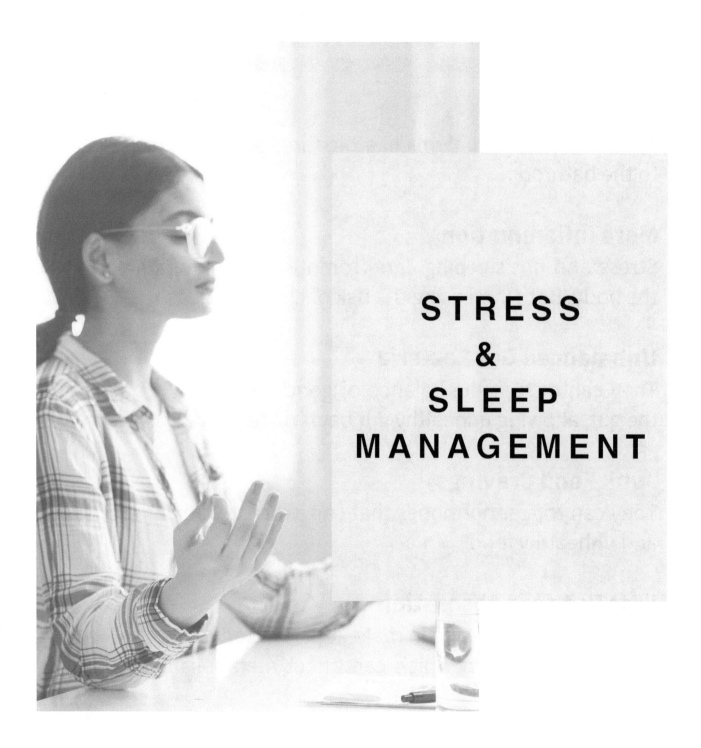

STRESS
&
SLEEP
MANAGEMENT

5 Ways Lack of Sleep and Stress Can Impact Gut Health

Stomach Issues
They can cause problems like bloating, gas, and trouble going to the bathroom.

More Inflammation
Stress and not sleeping can promote chronic inflammation in the body. Both increasing the risk of chronic disease.

Unbalanced Gut Bacteria
They can disrupt the balance of good and bad gut bacteria in the gut, allowing unhealthy gut bacteria to thrive.

Junk Food Cravings
They can trigger hormones that can promote cravings for sugar and unhealthy food.

Less Nutrient Absorption
Stress and poor sleep can make it harder for your gut to take in nutrients from food which can affect metabolism and weight management.

S.H.I.F.T. *Reflections*

I am grateful for:

1. _____
2. _____
3. _____

Things I can do to make this week great:

1. _____
2. _____
3. _____

Any Thoughts and Reflections

_____
_____
_____
_____
_____

Day 1

DATE

S.H.I.F.T. WELLNESS LOG

Sleep Time

Wake Up :   Go to Bed :

Stress Level

Fitness & Movement

Workout Activities

Total Minutes

Total Steps

Water Intake (cups)

Intestinal Health

Bowel Habits ☐

Probiotics ☐

Gut Detox ☐

Healthy Eating

Breakfast :

Lunch :

Dinner :

Snacks :

Each meal should include protein, a variety of vegetables, whole grains, healthy fats, and a serving of fruit for balanced nutrition at least 80% of the time.

Today I am feeling...

_____

_____

_____

_____

_____

_____

_____

_____

_____

Day 1
Focus: Stress & Sleep Management

> "I let go of chaos and confusion that are out
> my control that promote stress in my life."

S.H.I.F.T. Activity: Identify Stressors

- List 2 main stressors
- Identify what triggers your stress and how you currently handle it

_____

_____

_____

_____

_____

_____

Trust The Process: **Three great things that happened today**

_____

_____

_____

_____

_____

Day 2

DATE

S.H.I.F.T. WELLNESS LOG

Sleep Time

Wake Up :   Go to Bed :

Stress Level

Fitness & Movement

Workout Activities

Total Minutes

Total Steps

Water Intake (cups)

Intestinal Health

Bowel Habits ☐

Probiotics ☐

Gut Detox ☐

Healthy Eating

Breakfast :

Lunch :

Dinner :

Snacks :

Each meal should include protein, a variety of vegetables, whole grains, healthy fats, and a serving of fruit for balanced nutrition at least 80% of the time.

Today I am feeling...

_____

_____

_____

_____

_____

_____

_____

_____

_____

Day 2
Focus: Stress & Sleep Management

"I concentrate on aspects I can manage in a healthy manner to lower my body's stress levels."

S.H.I.F.T. Activity: Identify Stressors

- Set aside time to reflect on your day and consider what events or thoughts triggered stress. Document specific instances when you felt stressed, including the time, place, people involved, and how you responded.

_____

_____

_____

_____

Trust The Process: **Three great things that happened today**

_____

_____

_____

_____

Day 3

DATE

S.H.I.F.T. WELLNESS LOG

Sleep Time

Wake Up :   Go to Bed :

Stress Level

Fitness & Movement

Workout Activities

Total Minutes

Total Steps

Water Intake (cups)

Intestinal Health

Bowel Habits ☐

Probiotics ☐

Gut Detox ☐

Healthy Eating

Breakfast :

Lunch :

Dinner :

Snacks :

Each meal should include protein, a variety of vegetables, whole grains, healthy fats, and a serving of fruit for balanced nutrition at least 80% of the time.

Today I am feeling...

_____

_____

_____

_____

_____

_____

_____

_____

Day 3
Focus: Stress & Sleep Management

> "I release any negative beliefs or patterns
> that may be affecting my gut health."

S.H.I.F.T. Activity: Practice Self-Compassion

- Practice self-kindness and mindfulness to reduce self-criticism and increase emotional resilience. Give yourself grace in this process!
- Engage in self-compassion meditations or journaling exercises.

_____

_____

_____

_____

_____

Trust The Process: **Three great things that happened today**

_____

_____

_____

_____

_____

_____

Day 4

S.H.I.F.T. WELLNESS LOG

Sleep Time

Wake Up :   Go to Bed :

Stress Level

Fitness & Movement

Workout Activities

Total Minutes

Total Steps

Water Intake (cups)

Intestinal Health

Bowel Habits ☐

Probiotics ☐

Gut Detox ☐

Healthy Eating

Breakfast :

Lunch :

Dinner :

Snacks :

Each meal should include protein, a variety of vegetables, whole grains, healthy fats, and a serving of fruit for balanced nutrition at least 80% of the time.

Today I am feeling...

_____

_____

_____

_____

_____

_____

_____

_____

Day 4
Focus: Practice Relaxation Techniques

> "I release any tension or stress held in my gut, allowing for deep relaxation and healing."

S.H.I.F.T. Activity: Breathing

Try deep breathing exercises (10 minutes) throughout the day.
How do you feel?

_____

_____

_____

_____

_____

_____

Trust The Process: Three great things that happened today

_____

_____

_____

_____

_____

Day 5

S.H.I.F.T. WELLNESS LOG

Sleep Time

Wake Up :   Go to Bed :

Stress Level

Fitness & Movement

Workout Activities

Total Minutes

Total Steps

Water Intake (cups)

Intestinal Health

Bowel Habits ☐

Probiotics ☐

Gut Detox ☐

Healthy Eating

Breakfast :

Lunch :

Dinner :

Snacks :

Each meal should include protein, a variety of vegetables, whole grains, healthy fats, and a serving of fruit for balanced nutrition at least 80% of the time.

Today I am feeling...

_____

_____

_____

_____

_____

_____

_____

_____

Day 5
Focus: Practice Relaxation Techniques

"I trust in the natural healing abilities of my gut
and support it by incorporating techniques
to manage stress. "

S.H.I.F.T. Activity: Meditation

Practice mindfulness meditation (15 minutes) throughout your day
How do you feel?

_____

_____

_____

_____

_____

_____

Trust The Process: Three great things that happened today

_____

_____

_____

_____

_____

_____

Day 6

S.H.I.F.T. WELLNESS LOG

Sleep Time

Wake Up :   Go to Bed :

Stress Level

Fitness & Movement

Workout Activities	Total Minutes	Total Steps
		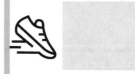

Water Intake (cups)

☐ ☐ ☐ ☐ ☐ ☐ ☐ ☐

Intestinal Health

Bowel Habits ☐

Probiotics ☐

Gut Detox ☐

Healthy Eating

Breakfast :

Lunch :

Dinner :

Snacks :

Each meal should include protein, a variety of vegetables, whole grains, healthy fats, and a serving of fruit for balanced nutrition at least 80% of the time.

Today I am feeling...

_____

_____

_____

_____

_____

_____

_____

_____

_____

Day 6
Focus: Practice Relaxation Techniques

"I connect with nature and spend time outdoors to promote a healthy gut-brain axis."

S.H.I.F.T. Activity: Nature Walk

Take a 20-minute nature walk. How do you feel?

_____

_____

_____

_____

_____

_____

Trust The Process: Three great things that happened today

_____

_____

_____

_____

_____

Day 7

DATE

S.H.I.F.T. WELLNESS LOG

Sleep Time

Wake Up :   Go to Bed :

Stress Level

Fitness & Movement

Workout Activities

Total Minutes

Total Steps

Water Intake (cups)

Intestinal Health

Bowel Habits	☐
Probiotics	☐
Gut Detox	☐

Healthy Eating

Breakfast :

Lunch :

Dinner :

Snacks :

Each meal should include protein, a variety of vegetables, whole grains, healthy fats, and a serving of fruit for balanced nutrition at least 80% of the time.

Today I am feeling...

_____

_____

_____

_____

_____

_____

_____

_____

_____

Day 7
Focus: Practice Relaxation Techniques

"I am open to exploring new ways to support
my gut health and well-being."

S.H.I.F.T. Activity: Favorite Hobby

Do a hobby you love *(for example: painting, reading, etc.)*
How do you feel?

_____

_____

_____

_____

_____

_____

Trust The Process: Three great things that happened today

_____

_____

_____

_____

_____

Day 8

S.H.I.F.T. WELLNESS LOG

Sleep Time

Wake Up :   Go to Bed :

Stress Level

Fitness & Movement

Workout Activities

Total Minutes

Total Steps

Water Intake (cups)

Intestinal Health

Bowel Habits ☐

Probiotics ☐

Gut Detox ☐

Healthy Eating

Breakfast :

Lunch :

Dinner :

Snacks :

Each meal should include protein, a variety of vegetables, whole grains, healthy fats, and a serving of fruit for balanced nutrition at least 80% of the time.

Today I am feeling...

_____

_____

_____

_____

_____

_____

_____

_____

Day 8
Focus: Sleep Improvement

**"I am promoting proper sleep
to support my body's healing capacity."**

S.H.I.F.T. Activity: Establish a Sleep Routine

- Attempt to be in bed by 10pm for at least 7 hours of sleep
- Steer clear of thoughts of anger or choas to enhance sleep quality

_____

_____

_____

_____

_____

Trust The Process: Three great things that happened today

_____

_____

_____

_____

_____

Day 9

S.H.I.F.T. WELLNESS LOG

Sleep Time

Wake Up :   Go to Bed :

Stress Level

Fitness & Movement

Workout Activities

Total Minutes

Total Steps

Water Intake (cups)

Intestinal Health

Bowel Habits	☐
Probiotics	☐
Gut Detox	☐

Healthy Eating

Breakfast :

Lunch :

Dinner :

Snacks :

Each meal should include protein, a variety of vegetables, whole grains, healthy fats, and a serving of fruit for balanced nutrition at least 80% of the time.

Today I am feeling...

_____

_____

_____

_____

_____

_____

_____

_____

_____

Day 9
Focus: Sleep Improvement

"I prioritize quality sleep, knowing it plays
a vital role in gut restoration and repair."

S.H.I.F.T. Activity: Enhance Sleep Quality

- Spend 15 minutes meditating and taking deep breaths before going to bed.
- Let go of negative and chaotic thoughts.

_____

_____

_____

_____

_____

_____

Trust The Process: Three great things that happened today

_____

_____

_____

_____

_____

Day 10

DATE

S.H.I.F.T. WELLNESS LOG

Sleep Time

Wake Up :   Go to Bed :

Stress Level

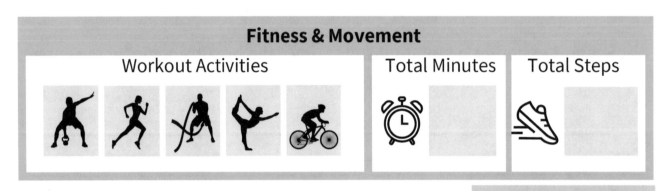

Fitness & Movement

Workout Activities

Total Minutes

Total Steps

Water Intake (cups)

Intestinal Health

Bowel Habits ☐

Probiotics ☐

Gut Detox ☐

Healthy Eating

Breakfast :

Lunch :

Dinner :

Snacks :

Each meal should include protein, a variety of vegetables, whole grains, healthy fats, and a serving of fruit for balanced nutrition at least 80% of the time.

Today I am feeling...

_____

_____

_____

_____

_____

_____

_____

_____

Day 10
Focus: Sleep Improvement

"With every night of quality sleep, I balance my microbiome, reduce inflammation, and support a healthy and resilient digestive system."

S.H.I.F.T. Activity: Avoid Sugar Before Bedtime

- Be sure dinner and/or night time snack is high in protein
- Turn phone notifications off at bedtime to promote uninterrupted sleep.

_____

_____

_____

_____

_____

Trust The Process: **Three great things that happened today**

_____

_____

_____

_____

_____

Day 11

DATE

S.H.I.F.T. WELLNESS LOG

Sleep Time

Wake Up :   Go to Bed :

Stress Level

Fitness & Movement

Workout Activities

Total Minutes

Total Steps

Water Intake (cups)

Intestinal Health

Bowel Habits ☐

Probiotics ☐

Gut Detox ☐

Healthy Eating

Breakfast :

Lunch :

Dinner :

Snacks :

Each meal should include protein, a variety of vegetables, whole grains, healthy fats, and a serving of fruit for balanced nutrition at least 80% of the time.

Today I am feeling...

Day 11
Focus: Create a Sleep-Friendly Environment

*"I am in tune with my body's unique needs
and adjust my lifestyle accordingly."*

S.H.I.F.T. Activity:

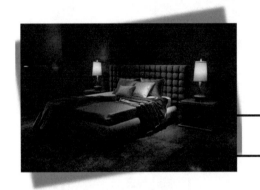

Sleep Environment

Make your bedroom dark and cool.

_____

_____

_____

_____

_____

_____

Trust The Process: **Three great things that happened today**

_____

_____

_____

_____

_____

_____

Day 12

DATE

S.H.I.F.T. WELLNESS LOG

Sleep Time

Wake Up :   Go to Bed :

Stress Level

Fitness & Movement

Workout Activities

Total Minutes

Total Steps

Water Intake (cups)

Intestinal Health

Bowel Habits ☐

Probiotics ☐

Gut Detox ☐

Healthy Eating

Breakfast :

Lunch :

Dinner :

Snacks :

Each meal should include protein, a variety of vegetables, whole grains, healthy fats, and a serving of fruit for balanced nutrition at least 80% of the time.

Today I am feeling...

_____

_____

_____

_____

_____

_____

_____

_____

_____

Day 12
Focus: Create a Sleep-Friendly Environment

"I cultivate a positive mindset, knowing that
my thoughts and emotions impact my gut health."

S.H.I.F.T. Activity: Sleep Environment

Use a white noise machine or earplugs if needed.

_____

_____

_____

_____

_____

_____

Trust The Process: Three great things that happened today

_____

_____

_____

_____

_____

_____

Day 13

S.H.I.F.T. WELLNESS LOG

Sleep Time

Wake Up :   Go to Bed :

Stress Level

Fitness & Movement

Workout Activities

Total Minutes

Total Steps

Water Intake (cups)

Intestinal Health

Bowel Habits ☐

Probiotics ☐

Gut Detox ☐

Healthy Eating

Breakfast :

Lunch :

Dinner :

Snacks :

Each meal should include protein, a variety of vegetables, whole grains, healthy fats, and a serving of fruit for balanced nutrition at least 80% of the time.

Today I am feeling...

_____

_____

_____

_____

_____

_____

_____

_____

Day 13
Focus: Create a Sleep-Friendly Environment

"As I rest, my gut heals and restores, allowing my digestion to function optimally and my health to thrive."

S.H.I.F.T. Activity:

Sleep Environment

Invest in a comfortable mattress and pillows.

_____

_____

_____

_____

_____

_____

Trust The Process: **Three great things that happened today**

_____

_____

_____

_____

_____

_____

Day 14

DATE

S.H.I.F.T. WELLNESS LOG

Sleep Time

Wake Up :   Go to Bed :

Stress Level

Fitness & Movement

Workout Activities

Total Minutes

Total Steps

Water Intake (cups)

Intestinal Health

Bowel Habits ☐

Probiotics ☐

Gut Detox ☐

Healthy Eating

Breakfast :

Lunch :

Dinner :

Snacks :

Each meal should include protein, a variety of vegetables, whole grains, healthy fats, and a serving of fruit for balanced nutrition at least 80% of the time.

Today I am feeling...

_____

_____

_____

_____

_____

_____

_____

_____

Day 14
Focus: Create a Sleep-Friendly Environment

> "I am mindful of the impact of poor sleep on my gut and take steps to manage it effectively."

S.H.I.F.T. Activity:

Sleep Environment

Avoid caffeine and heavy meals before bed.

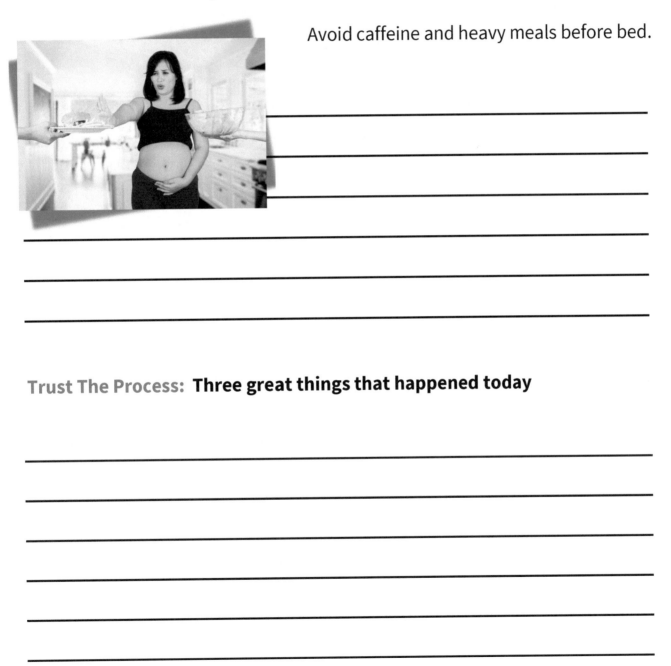

_____

_____

_____

_____

_____

_____

Trust The Process: **Three great things that happened today**

_____

_____

_____

_____

_____

_____

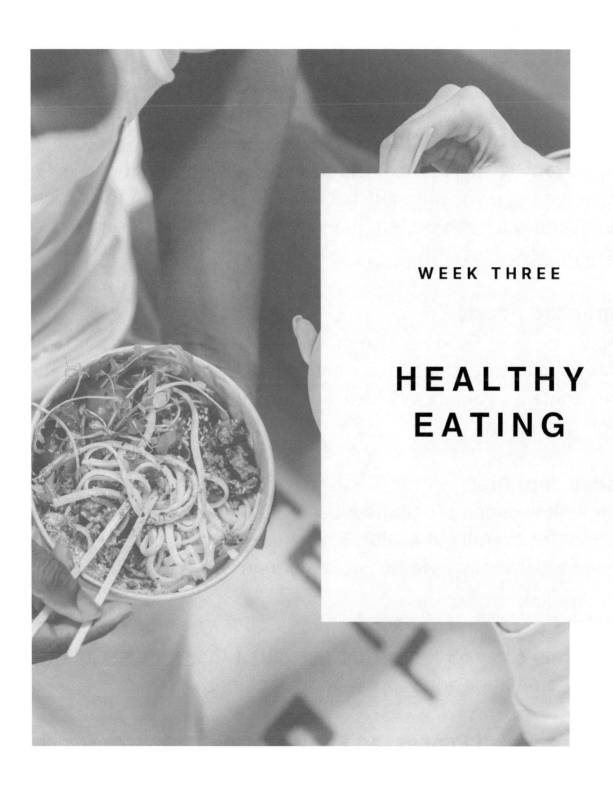

WEEK THREE

HEALTHY EATING

5 Ways Healthy Eating Promotes Healthy Gut Bacteria

Fruit, Vegetables, & Whole Grains

It's important to include to include fiber and vegetables in every meal to feed your healthy gut bacteria. Aim for 28 grams of fiber each day, include lean protein in every meal, and eat 5 servings of fruits and vegetables daily.

Fermented Foods

Trying Fermented Foods is also great. Adding yogurt to your daily diet and your smoothies is an easy way. Kefir, sauerkraut, and kimchi contain probiotics, which are also beneficial bacteria that support gut health.

Broaden Your Diet

Eating various foods promotes a diverse gut microbiome, which is important for overall gut health. Take a look at your diet by doing a 24-hour food inventory of what you eat for an entire day!

Healthy Fats

Foods rich in omega-3 fatty acids, like fatty fish and nuts, can help reduce inflammation and support good bacteria.

Limit Sugar and Processed Foods

Reducing sugar and processed foods can help prevent the growth of harmful bacteria and support a healthier gut environment. Choose organic foods whenever possible!

S.H.I.F.T. *Reflections*

I am grateful for:

1. _____

2. _____

3. _____

Things I can do to make this week great:

1. _____

2. _____

3. _____

Any Thoughts and Reflections

_____

_____

_____

_____

_____

Day 15

S.H.I.F.T. WELLNESS LOG

Sleep Time

Wake Up :   Go to Bed :

Stress Level

Fitness & Movement

Workout Activities

Total Minutes

Total Steps

Water Intake (cups)

☐ ☐ ☐ ☐ ☐ ☐ ☐ ☐

Intestinal Health

Bowel Habits ☐

Probiotics ☐

Gut Detox ☐

Healthy Eating

Breakfast :

Lunch :

Dinner :

Snacks :

Each meal should include protein, a variety of vegetables, whole grains, healthy fats, and a serving of fruit for balanced nutrition at least 80% of the time.

Today I am feeling...

_____

_____

_____

_____

_____

_____

_____

_____

_____

Day 15
Focus: Plan Balanced Meals

> "I choose to fuel my body with nourishing
> foods that support my gut health."

MON	BREAKFAST	DINNER
	LUNCH	SNACK
TUE	BREAKFAST	DINNER
	LUNCH	SNACK
WED	BREAKFAST	DINNER
	LUNCH	SNACK
THUR	BREAKFAST	DINNER
	LUNCH	SNACK
FRI	BREAKFAST	DINNER
	LUNCH	SNACK
SAT	BREAKFAST	DINNER
	LUNCH	SNACK
SUN	BREAKFAST	DINNER
	LUNCH	SNACK

S.H.I.F.T. Activity:

Meal Plan

Include a variety of fruits,
vegetables, lean proteins,
and whole grains.
Plan your meals for the week.

_____

_____

_____

_____

_____

_____

_____

_____

_____

_____

_____

_____

_____

_____

_____

_____

_____

_____

Day 16

DATE

S.H.I.F.T. WELLNESS LOG

Sleep Time

Wake Up :   Go to Bed :

Stress Level

Fitness & Movement

Workout Activities

Total Minutes

Total Steps

Water Intake (cups)

Intestinal Health

Bowel Habits ☐
Probiotics ☐
Gut Detox ☐

Healthy Eating

Breakfast :

Lunch :

Dinner :

Snacks :

Each meal should include protein, a variety of vegetables, whole grains, healthy fats, and a serving of fruit for balanced nutrition at least 80% of the time.

Today I am feeling...

_____

_____

_____

_____

_____

_____

_____

_____

Day 16
Focus: Plan Balanced Meals

> "I embrace a diverse and colorful diet
> to promote a healthy gut microbiome."

S.H.I.F.T. Activity: Meal Plan

Add at least one new activity to your meal plan each day for the next 30 days.

Add some protein	Use whole grains	Fill up on fiber	Don't skip dinner	Try a new veggie
Eat fruits first	Skip dessert	Eliminate sugar	Upgrade your snack	No ice cream
Skip Soda	Mix up your protein	Drink more water	Cut out bad carbs	Eliminate alcohol
Don't skip breakfast	No fast food	Try leafy greens	Morning smoothie	Nutritious breakfast
Eliminate dairy	Avoid salt	Cook at home	Drink herbal tea	Eat vegetables
Snack on fresh fruits	Eliminate coffee	Eat more veggies	Eliminate MSG	Go gluten free

Day 17

DATE

S.H.I.F.T. WELLNESS LOG

Sleep Time

Wake Up :   Go to Bed :

Stress Level

Fitness & Movement

Workout Activities

Total Minutes

Total Steps

Water Intake (cups)

Intestinal Health

Bowel Habits ☐

Probiotics ☐

Gut Detox ☐

Healthy Eating

Breakfast :

Lunch :

Dinner :

Snacks :

Each meal should include protein, a variety of vegetables, whole grains, healthy fats, and a serving of fruit for balanced nutrition at least 80% of the time.

Today I am feeling...

_____

_____

_____

_____

_____

_____

_____

_____

Day 17
Focus: Plan Balanced Meals

"I trust in the power of fermented foods to enhance my gut health."

S.H.I.F.T. Activity: Meal Planning

How do you feel your meal planning has helped you thus far?

_____

_____

_____

_____

_____

Trust The Process: Three great things that happened today

_____

_____

_____

_____

_____

Day 18

S.H.I.F.T. WELLNESS LOG

Sleep Time

Wake Up :   Go to Bed :

Stress Level

Fitness & Movement

Workout Activities	Total Minutes	Total Steps

Water Intake (cups)

Intestinal Health

Bowel Habits ☐

Probiotics ☐

Gut Detox ☐

Healthy Eating

Breakfast :

Lunch :

Dinner :

Snacks :

Each meal should include protein, a variety of vegetables, whole grains, healthy fats, and a serving of fruit for balanced nutrition at least 80% of the time.

Today I am feeling...

_____

_____

_____

_____

_____

_____

_____

_____

Day 18
Focus: Hydrate Properly

> "I nourish my body by drinking water daily, keeping myself hydrated and energized."

S.H.I.F.T. Activity:

Drink at least 8 glasses of water a day. Reduce sugary drinks and caffeine intake.

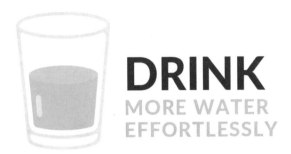

How many 8oz cups did you drink today?

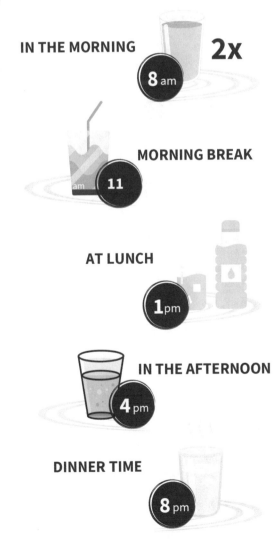

IN THE MORNING **2x** **8** am

MORNING BREAK **11** am

AT LUNCH **1** pm

IN THE AFTERNOON **4** pm

DINNER TIME **8** pm

Day 19

S.H.I.F.T. WELLNESS LOG

Sleep Time

Wake Up :   Go to Bed :

Stress Level

Fitness & Movement

Workout Activities

Total Minutes	Total Steps

Water Intake (cups)

Intestinal Health

Bowel Habits ☐
Probiotics ☐
Gut Detox ☐

Healthy Eating

Breakfast :

Lunch :

Dinner :

Snacks :

Each meal should include protein, a variety of vegetables, whole grains, healthy fats, and a serving of fruit for balanced nutrition at least 80% of the time.

Today I am feeling...

_____

_____

_____

_____

_____

_____

_____

_____

Day 19
Focus: Hydrate Properly

> "Every sip of water I take revitalizes my body and supports my overall well-being."

S.H.I.F.T. Activity: Try Infused Water

Drink at least 8 glasses of water a day. Avoid drinking a lot of water with meals to promote healthy digestion. Excess water with meals can dilute digestive enzyme.

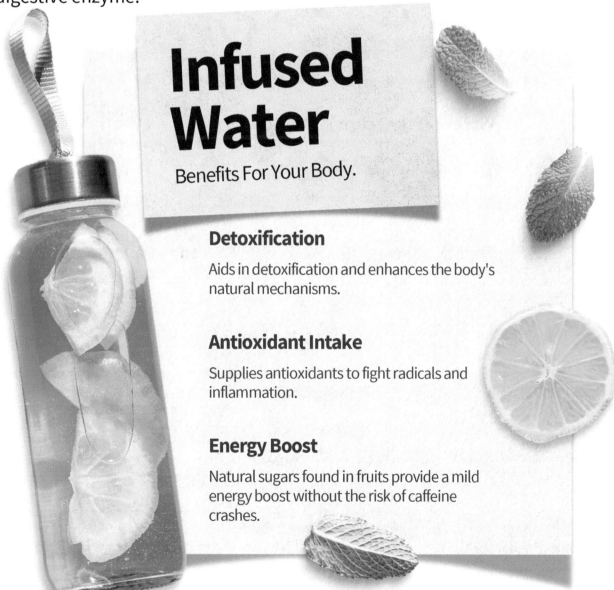

Infused Water

Benefits For Your Body.

Detoxification

Aids in detoxification and enhances the body's natural mechanisms.

Antioxidant Intake

Supplies antioxidants to fight radicals and inflammation.

Energy Boost

Natural sugars found in fruits provide a mild energy boost without the risk of caffeine crashes.

Day 20

DATE

S.H.I.F.T. WELLNESS LOG

Sleep Time

Wake Up :   Go to Bed :

Stress Level

Fitness & Movement

Workout Activities

Total Minutes

Total Steps

Water Intake (cups)

Intestinal Health

Bowel Habits ☐

Probiotics ☐

Gut Detox ☐

Healthy Eating

Breakfast :

Lunch :

Dinner :

Snacks :

Each meal should include protein, a variety of vegetables, whole grains, healthy fats, and a serving of fruit for balanced nutrition at least 80% of the time.

Today I am feeling...

_____

_____

_____

_____

_____

_____

_____

_____

Day 20
Focus: Hydrate Properly

"I prioritize hydration because it fuels my body, enhances my energy, and keeps me healthy."

S.H.I.F.T. Activity: Drink More Water

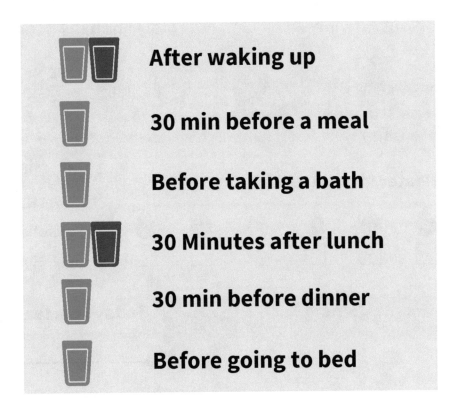

After waking up

30 min before a meal

Before taking a bath

30 Minutes after lunch

30 min before dinner

Before going to bed

1 Water is vital for keeping the body functioning properly.

2 Drinking water promotes more elastic and radiant skin.

3 Proper hydration enhances concentration and mental clarity.

4 Water helps control appetite and calorie intake.

Day 21

DATE

S.H.I.F.T. WELLNESS LOG

Sleep Time

Wake Up :   Go to Bed :

Stress Level

Fitness & Movement

Workout Activities

Total Minutes

Total Steps

Water Intake (cups)

Intestinal Health

Bowel Habits ☐

Probiotics ☐

Gut Detox ☐

Healthy Eating

Breakfast :

Lunch :

Dinner :

Snacks :

Each meal should include protein, a variety of vegetables, whole grains, healthy fats, and a serving of fruit for balanced nutrition at least 80% of the time.

Today I am feeling...

_____

_____

_____

_____

_____

_____

_____

_____

Day 21
Focus: Hydrate Properly

"By drinking water regularly, I give my body the hydration it needs to function at its best."

S.H.I.F.T. Activity: Drink More Water

How do you feel after incorporating more water into your diet?

_____

_____

_____

_____

_____

Trust The Process: **Three great things that happened today**

_____

_____

_____

_____

_____

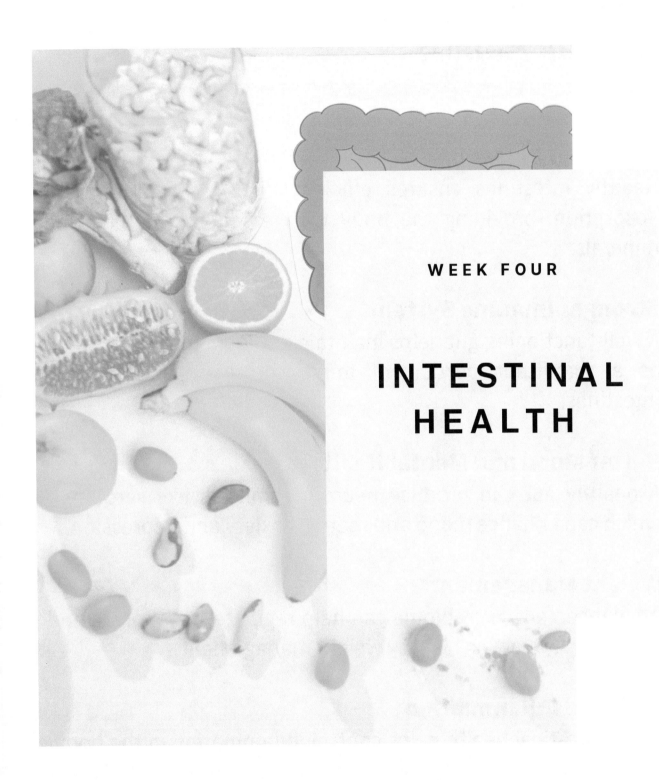

WEEK FOUR

INTESTINAL HEALTH

5 Ways Intestinal Health Promotes Overall Health

Improved Digestion

Healthy intestines ensures efficient digestion and nutrient absorption, providing the body with essential vitamins and minerals.

Stronger Immune System

A well-functioning gut helps maintain a strong immune system, as a significant portion of immune cells resides in the intestines.

Better Mood and Mental Health

A healthy gut can produce neurotransmitters like serotonin, which can enhance mood and reduce anxiety and depression.

Weight Management

A balanced gut microbiome can help regulate metabolism and appetite, supporting healthy weight management.

Reduced Inflammation

Good intestinal health helps control inflammation in the body, which can lower the risk of chronic diseases like heart disease and diabetes.

S.H.I.F.T. *Reflections*

I am grateful for:

1. _____

2. _____

3. _____

Things I can do to make this week great:

1. _____

2. _____

3. _____

Any Thoughts and Reflections

_____

_____

_____

_____

_____

Day 22

S.H.I.F.T. WELLNESS LOG

Sleep Time

Wake Up :   Go to Bed :

Stress Level

Fitness & Movement

Workout Activities

Total Minutes	Total Steps

Water Intake (cups)

Intestinal Health

Bowel Habits ☐

Probiotics ☐

Gut Detox ☐

Healthy Eating

Breakfast :

Lunch :

Dinner :

Snacks :

Each meal should include protein, a variety of vegetables, whole grains, healthy fats, and a serving of fruit for balanced nutrition at least 80% of the time.

Today I am feeling...

_____

_____

_____

_____

_____

_____

_____

_____

Day 22
Focus: Intestinal Health

"I nourish my gut with prebiotic-rich foods, supporting the growth of beneficial bacteria."

S.H.I.F.T. Activity: Introduce Probiotic Foods

- Add yogurt, kefir, and/or our holistic probiotic supplement to your diet!
- Eat fiber-rich foods like fruits, vegetables, and whole grains.

_____

_____

_____

_____

_____

Trust The Process: Three great things that happened today

_____

_____

_____

_____

_____

Day 23

DATE

S.H.I.F.T. WELLNESS LOG

Sleep Time

Wake Up :   Go to Bed :

Stress Level

Fitness & Movement

Workout Activities

Total Minutes

Total Steps

Water Intake (cups)

Intestinal Health

Bowel Habits ☐

Probiotics ☐

Gut Detox ☐

Healthy Eating

Breakfast :

Lunch :

Dinner :

Snacks :

Each meal should include protein, a variety of vegetables, whole grains, healthy fats, and a serving of fruit for balanced nutrition at least 80% of the time.

Today I am feeling...

_____

_____

_____

_____

_____

_____

_____

_____

Day 23

Focus: Intestinal Health

"I honor the connection between my gut and immune system, supporting overall wellness."

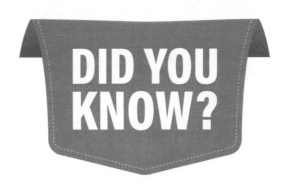

Gut Health has a big impact on inflammation in the body.

Your Gut is an influence and reflection on every cell, organ, and system in your body.

Leaky Gut occurs when the lining of the intestines becomes damaged allowing toxins and undigested food particles to enter the blood stream and trigger inflammation.

_____

_____

_____

Day 24

DATE

S.H.I.F.T. WELLNESS LOG

Sleep Time

Wake Up :   Go to Bed :

Stress Level

Fitness & Movement

Workout Activities	Total Minutes	Total Steps

Water Intake (cups)

Intestinal Health

Bowel Habits ☐
Probiotics ☐
Gut Detox ☐

Healthy Eating

Breakfast :

Lunch :

Dinner :

Snacks :

Each meal should include protein, a variety of vegetables, whole grains, healthy fats, and a serving of fruit for balanced nutrition at least 80% of the time.

Today I am feeling...

_____

_____

_____

_____

_____

_____

_____

_____

Day 24
Focus: Intestinal Health

"My Gut Health is an influence and reflection of my overall health and wellness."

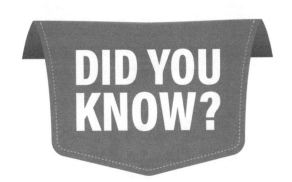

The Gut's effect on inflammation can promote chronic diseases like high blood pressure, diabetes, cardiovascular disease, and so much more.

- Continue on our holistic probotics with digestive enzymes & ginger
- Eat fiber-rich foods like fruits, vegetables, and whole grains.

_____

_____

_____

_____

_____

_____

Day 25

DATE

S.H.I.F.T. WELLNESS LOG

Sleep Time

Wake Up :   Go to Bed :

Stress Level

Fitness & Movement

Workout Activities

Total Minutes

Total Steps

Water Intake (cups)

Intestinal Health

Bowel Habits ☐

Probiotics ☐

Gut Detox ☐

Healthy Eating

Breakfast :

Lunch :

Dinner :

Snacks :

Each meal should include protein, a variety of vegetables, whole grains, healthy fats, and a serving of fruit for balanced nutrition at least 80% of the time.

Today I am feeling...

_____

_____

_____

_____

_____

_____

_____

_____

Day 25
Focus: Intestinal Health

> "I am patient and kind with myself
> as I embark on my gut wellness journey."

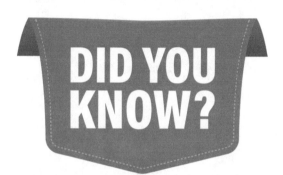

**Gut Health makes an impact on
your metabolism and weight management.**

At least 70% of our immune system is in our gut.

**Food sensitivities, bloating, and gas
are signs of an unhealthy gut.**

- Avoid processed foods and excess sugar.
- Eat fermented foods like sauerkraut or kimchi.

_____

_____

_____

_____

_____

_____

Day 26

S.H.I.F.T. WELLNESS LOG

Sleep Time

Wake Up :   Go to Bed :

Stress Level

Fitness & Movement

Workout Activities

Total Minutes

Total Steps

Water Intake (cups)

Intestinal Health

Bowel Habits ☐

Probiotics ☐

Gut Detox ☐

Healthy Eating

Breakfast :

Lunch :

Dinner :

Snacks :

Each meal should include protein, a variety of vegetables, whole grains, healthy fats, and a serving of fruit for balanced nutrition at least 80% of the time.

Today I am feeling...

_____

_____

_____

_____

_____

_____

_____

_____

_____

Day 26
Focus: Maintain Gut Health

"I practice gratitude for my gut's role in maintaining my overall health."

S.H.I.F.T. Activity: Support Optimal Digestion

- Be sure drink 8 glasses of water daily
- Stay away from cold water during meals because it can slow down digestion

_____

_____

_____

_____

_____

Trust The Process: Three great things that happened today

_____

_____

_____

_____

_____

Day 27

S.H.I.F.T. WELLNESS LOG

Sleep Time

Wake Up :   Go to Bed :

Stress Level

Fitness & Movement

Workout Activities

Total Minutes

Total Steps

Water Intake (cups)

Intestinal Health

Bowel Habits ☐

Probiotics ☐

Gut Detox ☐

Healthy Eating

Breakfast :

Lunch :

Dinner :

Snacks :

Each meal should include protein, a variety of vegetables, whole grains, healthy fats, and a serving of fruit for balanced nutrition at least 80% of the time.

Today I am feeling...

_____

_____

_____

_____

_____

_____

_____

_____

Day 27
Focus: Intestinal Health

"I am open to receiving guidance
and knowledge about gut health."

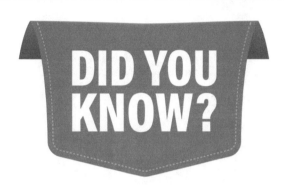

Inflammation from poor gut health can influence and affect mood, anxiety, and depression.

Hormones in your gut can influence your cravings for carbs and sugar

Your healthy gut bacteria secrete a hormone called GLP-1, which lowers the risk of obesity, diabetes, metabolic syndrome while also reducing inflammation.

_____

_____

_____

_____

_____

Day 28

DATE

S.H.I.F.T. WELLNESS LOG

Sleep Time

Wake Up :   Go to Bed :

Stress Level

Fitness & Movement

Workout Activities

Total Minutes

Total Steps

Water Intake (cups)

Intestinal Health

Bowel Habits ☐

Probiotics ☐

Gut Detox ☐

Healthy Eating

Breakfast :

Lunch :

Dinner :

Snacks :

Each meal should include protein, a variety of vegetables, whole grains, healthy fats, and a serving of fruit for balanced nutrition at least 80% of the time.

Today I am feeling...

_____

_____

_____

_____

_____

_____

_____

_____

_____

Day 28
Focus: Intestinal Health

> "I trust in the body's innate ability
> to heal and restore gut balance."

S.H.I.F.T. Activity: Promote Healthy Digestion

- Chew food thoroughly to support healthy digestion
- Avoid eating on the go to support healthy digestion

_____

_____

_____

_____

_____

Trust The Process: Three great things that happened today

_____

_____

_____

_____

_____

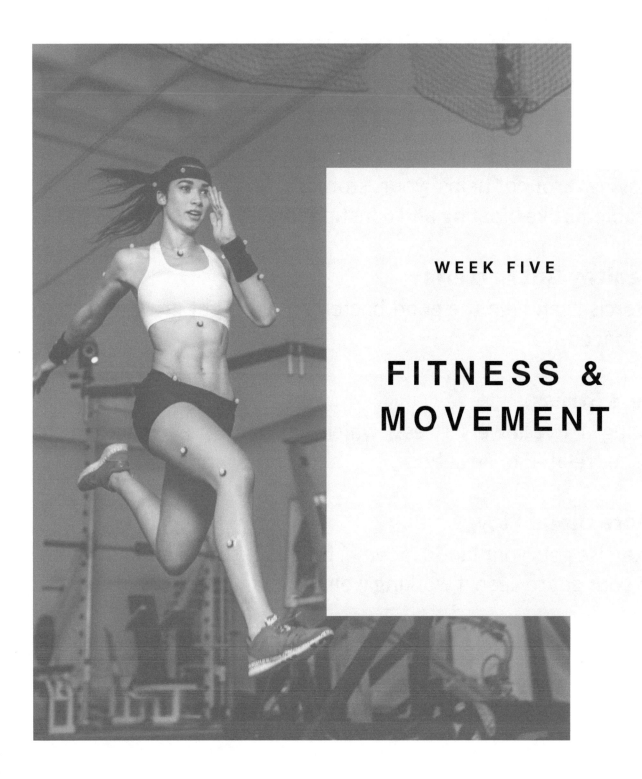

WEEK FIVE

FITNESS & MOVEMENT

5 Ways Fitness and Movement Help To Keep Your Gut Healthy

Better Digestion

Moving around helps your stomach work better, reducing problems like bloating and constipation.

Healthy Gut Bacteria

Exercise can help the good bacteria in your gut grow and stay balanced.

Less Stress

Being active lowers stress, which can help prevent stomach issues related to anxiety.

More Blood Flow

Exercise gets your blood moving, bringing oxygen and nutrients to your gut to keep it working well.

Healthy Weight

Staying active helps you maintain a healthy weight, which is good for your gut and can prevent digestive problems.

S.H.I.F.T. *Reflections*

I am grateful for:

1. _____

2. _____

3. _____

Things I can do to make this week great:

1. _____

2. _____

3. _____

Any Thoughts and Reflections

_____

_____

_____

_____

_____

Day 29

DATE

S.H.I.F.T. WELLNESS LOG

Sleep Time

Wake Up :   Go to Bed :

Stress Level

Fitness & Movement

Workout Activities

Total Minutes

Total Steps

Water Intake (cups)

Intestinal Health

Bowel Habits ☐

Probiotics ☐

Gut Detox ☐

Healthy Eating

Breakfast :

Lunch :

Dinner :

Snacks :

Each meal should include protein, a variety of vegetables, whole grains, healthy fats, and a serving of fruit for balanced nutrition at least 80% of the time.

Today I am feeling...

_____

_____

_____

_____

_____

_____

_____

_____

Day 29
Focus: Fitness Routine

"I prioritize regular physical activity to support gut motility and overall digestive health."

S.H.I.F.T. Activity: Start a Fitness Routine

- Set aside 30 minutes for physical activity.
- Choose activities you enjoy (walking, cycling, swimming).

_____

_____

_____

_____

_____

_____

Trust The Process: **Three great things that happened today**

_____

_____

_____

_____

_____

Day 30

DATE

S.H.I.F.T. WELLNESS LOG

Sleep Time

Wake Up :   Go to Bed :

Stress Level

😊 🙂 😐 🙁 😭

Fitness & Movement

Workout Activities

Total Minutes

Total Steps

Water Intake (cups)

Intestinal Health

Bowel Habits ☐

Probiotics ☐

Gut Detox ☐

Healthy Eating

Breakfast :

Lunch :

Dinner :

Snacks :

Each meal should include protein, a variety of vegetables, whole grains, healthy fats, and a serving of fruit for balanced nutrition at least 80% of the time.

Today I am feeling...

_____

_____

_____

_____

_____

_____

_____

_____

Day 30
Focus: Mix It Up

"I am committed to maintaining a lifelong commitment to gut wellness, knowing it is the foundation of my health."

S.H.I.F.T. Activity: Mix It Up

- Try different types of exercise: strength training, cardio, yoga.
- Aim for at least 150 minutes of moderate exercise per week.

_____

_____

_____

_____

_____

_____

Trust The Process: **Three great things that happened today**

_____

_____

_____

_____

_____

_____

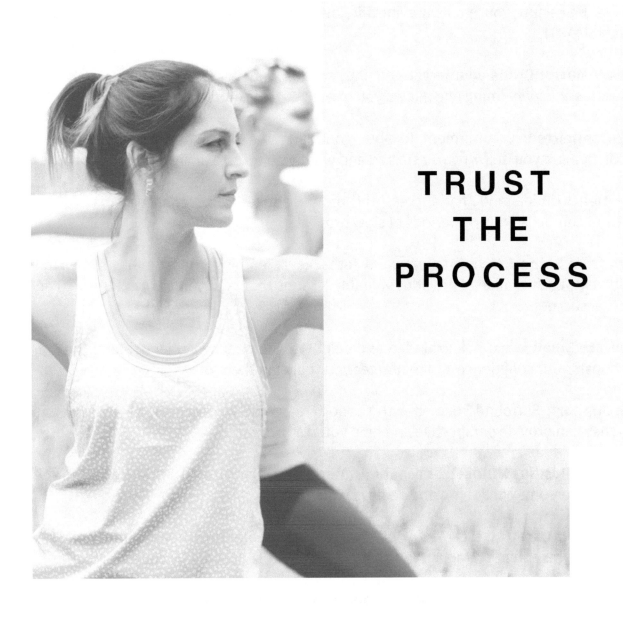

TRUST
THE
PROCESS

Trusting The Process

Trusting the process involves having faith in the journey towards a goal, despite not always seeing immediate results or understanding every step along the way. Here are some strategies to help you trust the process:

Set Clear Goals: Knowing what you are working towards helps keep you motivated and focused. Make sure your goals are specific, measurable, achievable, relevant, and time-bound (SMART).

Break It Down: Divide your larger goal into smaller, manageable tasks. This makes the process less overwhelming and allows you to see progress more clearly.

Stay Committed: Commitment to your goals and the process of achieving them is crucial. Remind yourself why you started and what you hope to achieve.

Be Patient: Understand that success and progress take time. Patience helps you stay calm and composed during periods of slow progress.

Learn from Setbacks: View failures and setbacks as learning opportunities rather than roadblocks. Each challenge provides valuable lessons that contribute to your growth and eventual success.

Celebrate Small Wins: Acknowledge and celebrate small achievements along the way. This boosts your confidence and reinforces your belief in the process.

Seek Support: Surround yourself with supportive people who encourage and motivate you. They can provide perspective and help you stay on track.

Maintain a Positive Mindset: Stay optimistic and keep a positive attitude. Believe in your ability to overcome challenges and achieve your goals.

Practice Self-Care: Take care of your physical and mental health. A healthy body and mind are better equipped to handle stress and stay focused on the journey.

Trusting the process is about having confidence in your ability to achieve your goals and recognizing that each step, no matter how small, is a part of your path to success.

Date:

Focus: Trust Process

I discovered this about myself...

S.H.I.F.T. Activity: **Introspection Journaling**

_____

_____

_____

_____

_____

_____

_____

_____

_____

_____

_____

_____

_____

*There is a **SHIFT** in the wellness atmosphere.*
*This is a **Movement** to provoke an awareness and awakening*
*to the **Importance of Gut Health***
and its link to every organ, cell, and system in the body.

Meet Paula Richardson, RN, MSN, NP-C

TN Health Solutions, LLC

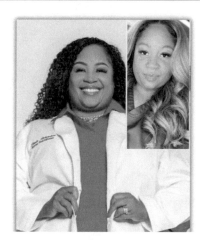

A highly accomplished individual who has made a significant impact in the field of healthcare and wellness. As the owner and founder of TopNotch Health Solutions, which began by offering free COVID-19 testing from the trunk of her 2020 Toyota Camry and served over 100,000 patients during the pandemic, she saw firsthand the impact of COVID-19 on those with chronic disease and obesity. By making a SHIFT in her own wellness, she was inspired to establish a renowned wellness center that takes an integrative and holistic approach to addressing obesity and metabolic health. A key focus of her center is on customized gut health, recognizing its vital role in overall well-being.

With an impressive nursing career spanning over 21 years, Paula is a dual board-certified advanced practice registered nurse. She holds certifications as a Family Nurse Practitioner, which she obtained from Georgia State University in 2012, and as an Adult Gerontology Acute Care Nurse Practitioner in 2017. She is further enhancing her education as a functional diagnostic practitioner. This extensive knowledge and expertise have positioned her as a trusted authority in the healthcare industry.

Driven by personal experiences with obesity, high blood pressure, and diabetes, Paula made a transformative shift from critical care to wellness using gut analysis and holistic gut wellness as a core component to identify healing opportunities. Motivated by her own journey towards better health, she has dedicated herself to helping others through her holistic approach to gut wellness & weight loss using functional testing to create individualized wellness plans. Her unique methods have positively impacted the lives of numerous clients, empowering them to achieve their health goals and live fulfilling lives. At her office in Riverdale, Georgia, Paula's wellness center has achieved a remarkable milestone with over 4,000 pounds lost collectively among her clients. This impressive accomplishment highlights the effectiveness of her unique and integrative approach to health and wellness, particularly in addressing obesity and metabolic issues holistic gut wellness as the core component.

Outside of her professional pursuits, Paula finds joy in her faith community and cherishes moments of meditation. She also maintains an active lifestyle, engaging in activities such as CrossFit to prioritize her own well-being. In her spare time, she enjoys the serenity of being by the river.

Paula Richardson is happily married to Robert Richardson, Jr., and together they are proud parents to four wonderful children. Her commitment to her family and her unwavering dedication to improving the lives of others make her an inspirational figure in both her personal and professional life.

Made in the USA
Columbia, SC
19 September 2024

42340790R10050